Cortisol Pump 101:
A Patient's Guide to Managing
The Cortisol Pumping Method

Copyright © 2021 Adrenal Alternatives Foundation © Winslow E. Dixon

CORTISOL PUMP

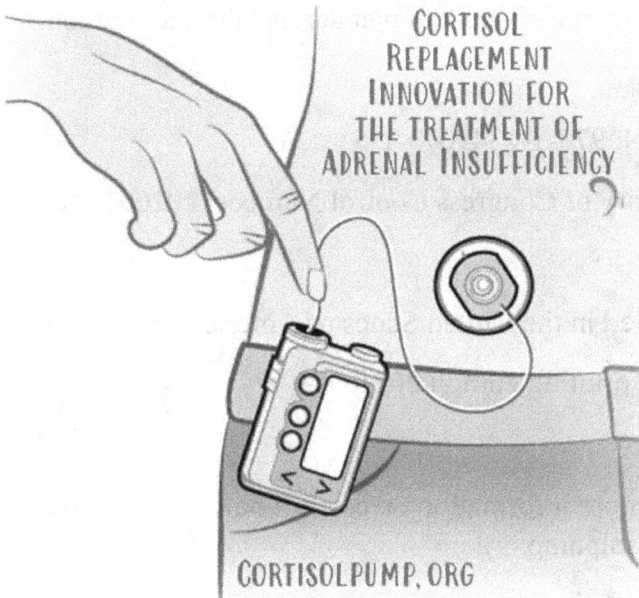

CORTISOL
REPLACEMENT
INNOVATION FOR
THE TREATMENT OF
ADRENAL INSUFFICIENCY

CORTISOLPUMP.ORG

This book was written from a patient's perspective and is not intended to give or replace medical care, advice or provide treatment of any medical condition.

ISBN: 978-1-7349073-1-5

Library of Congress Control Number: 2020919427

Printed in the United States of America.

First printing edition 2021

For more information on cortisol pumping visit the website: cortisolpump.org

Table of Contents

Chapter 1: Introduction

What is Adrenal Insufficiency?

Adrenal insufficiency is a condition where the adrenal glands fail to produce the proper amounts of steroid hormone(s). There are many different forms of adrenal disease, but the treatment for all forms requires cortisol replacement.

In a normal person, during situations of emotional or physical stress their body releases more cortisol. The excitement from a happy event, the sadness from a death of a loved one or the strain from exercising are examples of things that would cause the body to release more cortisol. In an adrenal insufficient person, this does not happen.

When someone has adrenal insufficiency, they are faced with the task of not only replacing a life-sustaining hormone, but also replicating a failed body system. Artificially managing cortisol is a complex task and is vital the quality of life. An adrenal patient's personal cortisol needs may differ from day to day depending on physical, emotional and environmental stressors.

Important Terms

Adrenal glands- Walnut shaped glands located on top of each kidney which produce cortisol. catecholamines, DHEA and androgenic steroids. The adrenal gland is comprised of:

1-Adrenal medulla- The inner part of an adrenal gland which controls hormones epinephrine (adrenaline) and norepinephrine (noradrenaline).

2- Adrenal cortex- The outer part of the gland that produces hormones such as cortisol and aldosterone.

Adrenal Insufficiency- Condition which results in the lack of cortisol production and can also result in lack of DHEA, aldosterone and disrupt the balance of the immune system, inflammation levels, endocrine hormones, electrolyte homeostasis, sodium and potassium levels and also can impact blood pressure and body temperature regulation. There are many forms of adrenal insufficiency.

Adrenocorticotropic hormone (ACTH) - Polypeptide tropic hormone which is crucial in the hypothalamic-pituitary-adrenal axis. ACTH is produced by the anterior pituitary gland and stimulates the adrenal glands to produce cortisol.

Aldosterone (ALD)- Mineralocorticoid hormone which regulates electrolyte balances by instructing the kidneys to release potassium and retain sodium. It also helps regulate blood pressure.

Antidiuretic Hormone (ADH)- Hormone also called arginine vasopressin which is made by the hypothalamus in the brain and stored in the posterior pituitary gland. ADH regulates the amount of water in the bloodstream by instructing the kidneys on how on much water to conserve.

Absorption- The ability of the body to absorb the infused mediation from the infusion pump site.

Bacteriostatic Water- Sterile water containing 0.9% benzyl alcohol that is used to reconstitute medication.

Basal Pattern- Delivery rates programmed into an infusion pump to dispense medication.

Basal Rate- Baseline amount of medication such as insulin or solu-cortef programmed into an infusion pump.

Bolus- Administration of an extra, single dose of medication such as insulin or solucortef. In the case of adrenal insufficiency, to bolus is to "updose" or take an extra amount of cortisol.

Bound Cortisol- Cortisol which is attached to a specific protein (CBG) is known as a bound cortisol. Metabolized cortisol evaluates how much cortisol is being made in total and cleared through the liver.

Cannula- A thin tube inserted into the body to administer medicine.

Catecholamines- Hormones such as dopamine, epinephrine (adrenaline) and norepinephrine (noradrenaline) that the adrenals produce in response to physical or emotional stress by increasing heart rate and blood pressure.

Cortisol– Glucocorticoid hormone: The body's stress hormone that is produced by the zona fasciculata. It helps control the body's use of fats, proteins and carbohydrates; suppresses inflammation, impacts blood pressure and blood sugar. It also controls the body's sleep/wake cycle and impacts the circadian rhythm.

Cortisol Binding Globulin (CBG)- Protein made by the liver which binds to cortisol and carries it through the body; also referred to as bound cortisol. 90-95 percent of cortisol in the body is in this form.

Circadian rhythm- The body's natural, internal process that regulates the sleep-wake cycle and repeats roughly every 24 hours. Circadian rhythms can be physical, mental, and behavioral patterns that follow a daily cycle. Cortisol is deeply crucial to circadian rhythm modulation.

CRH (corticotropin-releasing hormone)- A peptide hormone which the signals the pituitary synthesis of ACTH (Adrenocorticotropic hormone).

DHEA (dehydroepiandrosterone)- Hormone that aids in the production of androgens and estrogens (male and female sex hormones)

Day Curve- Lab test where a patient's blood serum cortisol levels are drawn every hour for twenty-four hours in order to calculate an appropriate baseline cortisol replacement dose and determine the patient's cortisol clearance rate.

Free Cortisol- Cortisol which is not attached to any protein known as free cortisol. Free cortisol reveals how much cortisol is free to bind to receptors and allows for assessment of the circadian rhythm. Free cortisol is sensed and regulated by the corticotrophin (CRH)–ACTH axis.

Fludrocortisone- Corticosteroid prescribed to treat salt wasting adrenogenital syndrome, POTS (postural hypotension) and some forms of adrenal insufficiency.

Glucocorticoids- Corticosteroid hormones that bind to glucocorticoid receptors and are part of the feedback mechanism in the immune system which reduces certain aspects of immune function, such as inflammation.

Infusion Pump- A medical device that dispenses medications such as insulin and solucortef into a patient's body at programable rates.

Infusion Set- The delivery device to that connects the infusion set into the body typically in the form of a needle inside a cannula which is placed into subcutaneous fatty tissue.

Infusion Site- Area of the body where the infusion pump cannula is inserted into subcutaneous fatty tissue to dispense medication such as insulin or solucortef.

Lipohypertrophy- Bump formed under the skin caused by accumulation of extra fat due to subcutaneous injections or infusion site placement.

Mg/DL- Milligrams per deciliter. A measurement that indicates the amount of a substance in a specific amount of blood.

Pod- Tubeless, waterproof infusion pump site.

Reservoir- Container that holds medication to be dispensed through the cannula via an infusion pump.

Saline- A mixture of sodium chloride and water used to clean wounds and reconstitute medication.

Salt Wasting- Term that refers to the medical condition where the adrenal glands make too little aldosterone, causing the body to be unable to retain enough sodium (salt) and resulting in too much sodium being lost in the urine.

Solu-Cortef- (Hydrocortisone sodium succinate) Glucocorticoid corticosteroid hormone medication that when mixed with saline or bacteriostatic water can be placed in an infusion pump and used to dispense 24/7 cortisol coverage in adrenal insufficient patients.

Sick Rates- Delivery rates set to administer elevated amounts of medication to manage sickness, injury or stress which require more medication such as solucortef.

Skin Prep- An alcohol swab or other cleaning solution used to sanitize the skin before injections or site placement.

Subcutaneous- Layer of skin directly below the dermis and epidermis.

Updose- To increase the dose of cortisol replacement medication according to physical, emotional or environmental stressors/needs to prevent low cortisol levels.

Mineralocorticoids- Corticosteroids that regulate electrolyte balance and fluid balance in the body. In salt wasting forms of adrenal disease, mineralocorticoid replacement is necessary. Medications such as fludrocortisone are used to supplement mineralocorticoid deficiency.

17-Hydroxyprogesterone- Endogenous progestogen steroid hormone related to progesterone which is critical in the biosynthesis of androgens, estrogens, glucocorticoids, and mineralocorticoids.

What is Cortisol Pumping?

The concept of Cortisol Pumping is the use of solu-cortef (inject-able version of cortisol when mixed with saline or bacteriostatic water) used in an insulin pump programmed to disperse cortisol according to the natural circadian rhythm by programming rates of delivery into the pump. This method bypasses the gastric passage and is able to deliver cortisol 24/7. With an infusion pump, an adrenal insufficient patient can receive a constant supply of cortisol and can lessen the instability experienced with oral steroid cortisol replacement. Side effects due to malabsorption can be decreased and patients have reported to have improved sleep, weight management and experience an overall improvement in their energy levels and sense of well-being. This method has also been shown to lessen the prevalence of adrenal crises and hospitalizations due to low cortisol.

Though this method is not a cure for adrenal disease, it is an option and a ray of hope for those who are struggling with quality of life.

Has it improved your quality of life?
52 responses

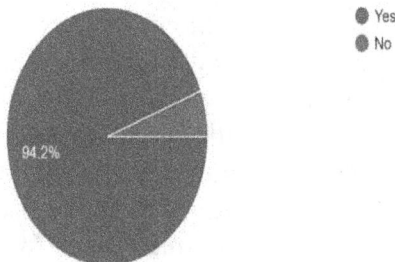

- Yes
- No

94.2%

11

According to a survey done by the Adrenal Alternatives Foundation, the data concluded that 94.2% of the 52 anonymous cortisol pumping patients reported that the cortisol pump had improved their quality of life.

Disclaimers:

The cortisol pumping method is not a cure for adrenal insufficiency and is not a "plug in and fix" treatment. Adrenal insufficiency is life threatening and must be properly treated.

The cortisol pumping method is not a replacement for an emergency cortisol injection.

Cortisol Pumping Myths

Myth #1 "It is not available."

The cortisol pumping method is a relatively unknown alternative treatment for adrenal insufficiency. Most doctors have never heard of it, but that does not mean it is not available. The use of infusion pumps to deliver medication is a common practice, mainly in the management of diabetes. However, the use of cortisol in infusion pumps is considered "off label" use. Cortisol pumping is available wherever infusion pumps are available. All you need is a doctor willing to manage your care, which involves he or she writing a prescription for an infusion pump, supplies and solu-cortef. Adrenal Alternatives Foundation works with patients internationally with cortisol pumping advocacy and we educate healthcare professionals all over the world on how to safely and effectively start the cortisol pumping method. We also work alongside other organizations to repurpose pumps and supplies to adrenal patients with our Pumps for Purpose program. Cortisol pumping is available internationally, wherever infusion pumps are available.

Myth #2 "My insurance won't cover it."

What your insurance will cover is completely dependent on your specific coverage plan and insurance company. If you are denied, you can file an appeal using the example appeal letter in the reference chapter of this book to contest your insurance company's denial. It is also an option to cash purchase a pump and supplies specifically from the company if you have a prescription from your overseeing physician.

Adrenal Alternatives Foundation has programs to help adrenal patients acquire pumps in a safe and legal manner. The foundation team also assists patients in filing insurance appeals has successfully battled countless insurance companies across the nation and can assist you in your fight for coverage.

Myth #3 "My doctor said no."

Finding a healthcare professional willing to work with this relatively unknown treatment option can be a challenge. You may have to "query" multiple physicians before you find one willing to manage your care on the cortisol pumping method. In order to achieve this, it is best to prepare a compelling case and provide it to the physician before your appointment. Send research on the cortisol pumping method (which can be found in the resources section of this book) and your health records to the physician before your appointment, so they are aware of your intentions beforehand. You can use the example pump proposal letter in the index to fill out with your information, explaining your diagnosis, failed treatments and desire to be on the pump. The doctor may or may not be receptive to your request and alerting them of your intentions beforehand may save you time, money and effort. Again, you may have to contact multiple physicians before finding one who is willing to manage the cortisol pumping method.

Cortisol Pumping FAQ

Is Cortisol Pumping FDA approved?

Adrenal Alternatives Foundation is actively working to gain FDA approval for the cortisol pumping method, but that involves clinical trials, patient studies and funding. We will achieve this one day, but until then, we are educating patients that FDA approval is not necessary to safely and legally begin cortisol pumping under the care of a licensed physician. Use of the infusion pump for adrenal insufficiency is legal and is medically considered "off label" use of the infusion pump technology.

Infusion pumps have long been approved for the administration of medications. According to the Department of Health and Human Services Centers for Medicare and Medicaid Services Medicare Coverage Issues Manual Section 60-14 A[1]: "6. Other uses of external infusion pumps are covered if the contractor's medical staff verifies the appropriateness of the therapy and of the prescribed pump for the individual patient."

In addition, according to the recently passed Right to Try Act[2], patients should have access to this treatment. The act states the following:

---

[1] "| Guidance Portal." U.S. Department of Health & Human Services Guidance Portal. 31 Dec. 2020. Web.

[2] FDA. "Right to Try Act." U.S. Food and Drug Administration. 14 Jan. 2020. Web.

(a) IN GENERAL.—Chapter V of the Federal Food, Drug, and Cosmetic Act is amended by inserting after section 561A (21 U.S.C. 360bbb–0) the following: "SEC. 561B. INVESTIGATION "SEC. 561B. INVESTIGATIONAL DRUGS FOR USE BY ELIGIBLE PATIENTS. "(a) DEFINITIONS.—For purposes of this section— "(1) the term 'eligible patient' means a patient— "(A) who has been diagnosed with a life-threatening disease or condition (as defined in section 312.81 of title 21, Code of Federal Regulations (or any successor regulations)); "(B) who has exhausted approved treatment options and is unable to participate in a clinical trial involving the eligible investigational drug, as certified by a physician, who— "(i) is in good standing with the physician's licensing organization or board; and "(ii) will not be compensated directly by the manufacturer for so certifying; and "(C) who has provided to the treating physician written informed consent regarding the eligible investigational drug, or, as applicable, on whose behalf a legally authorized representative of the patient has provided such consent."

According to the above legislation, adrenal patients meet the criteria for legal use of an infusion pump to administer glucocorticoid medication.

Is cortisol pumping safe?

Adrenal insufficiency requires adequate cortisol replacement in the form of steroid medications. With the cortisol pumping method, patients can bypass the gastric pathway and absorb their life-sustaining medication better. This treatment is revolutionary for hypermetabolizers and for those with gastro-intestinal problems or malabsorption issues. It provides 24/7 distribution of cortisol. The pump truly puts adrenal patients in control of their cortisol distribution in a way that steroid pills cannot. In situations of physical or emotional stress where "updosing" is needed, the pump can immediately administer a bolus, which is extra cortisol administered through the pump canula at the amount you select. Instead of having to wait for pills to metabolize, the cortisol can be absorbed faster and can help prevent adrenal crisis. Cortisol pumping is not a cure for adrenal insufficiency and is not a treatment that is right for everyone. If you are well managed on steroid replacement pills, being on the pump method may not be necessary to achieve quality of life.

Do I still need an emergency injection on the pumping method?

An adrenal crisis is defined as a life- threatening, medical emergency caused by insufficient levels of the hormone, cortisol. It will lead to death if left untreated and must be quickly addressed with the administration of an emergency cortisol injection. The pump is not a replacement for acute adrenal crisis care and patients should always carry an emergency injection and administer it immediately in the event of an adrenal crisis.

CORTISOLPUMP.ORG

500
400
300
200
100

1) 2) 3

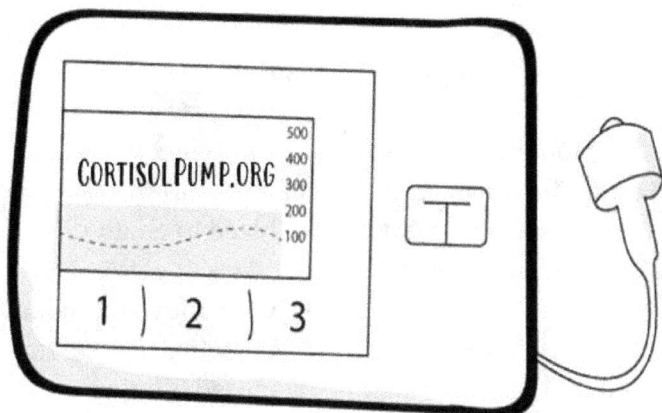

THE CORTISOL PUMP IS NOT A REPLACEMENT FOR AN EMERGENCY INJECTION TO TREAT AN ADRENAL CRISIS.

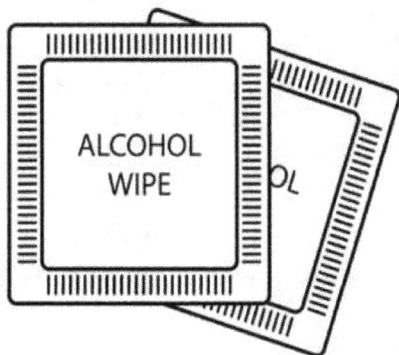

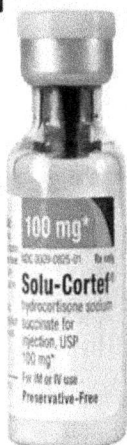

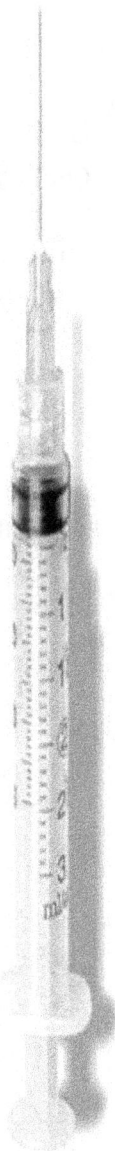

ALCOHOL WIPE

OL

100 mg*
NDC 0029-0825-01   Rx only
Solu-Cortef®
hydrocortisone sodium
succinate for
injection, USP
100 mg*
For IM or IV use
Preservative-Free

Chapter 2: Assessments

Evaluating Cortisol

Unfortunately, some cases of adrenal insufficiency are not diagnosed until after an adrenal crisis has occurred. An adrenal crisis is a serious event and will lead to death if left untreated. The body cannot sustain life without cortisol. Early detection can prevent damage to your body and make your prognosis with adrenal insufficiency better. Research[3] shows that adrenal disease patients diagnosed after an adrenal crisis are statistically less stable than those who are diagnosed never having an adrenal crisis. Getting the proper evaluation is essential to managing patient care with adrenal insufficiency. It is imperative that the correct tests are performed to assess adrenal function.

Adrenal Hormone Assessments[4]

ACTH Stimulation Test- When this test is done, your blood is drawn prior to injection of ACTH (Adrenocorticotropic hormone) then at timed intervals to test your adrenal's response to the ACTH. If your cortisol levels do not rise properly, you are then diagnosed with adrenal insufficiency.

Adrenal Antibodies Test- Also referred to as the 21-hydroxylase test which is used to investigate genetic causes

---

[3] Elshimy, Ghada. "Adrenal Crisis." StatPearls [Internet]. U.S. National Library of Medicine, 20 Nov. 2020. Web.
[4] "Diagnosing Adrenal Gland Disorders." Eunice Kennedy Shriver National Institute of Child Health and Human Development. U.S. Department of Health and Human Services, 31 Jan. 2017. Web.

of adrenal insufficiency such as congenital adrenal hyperplasia.

Catecholamine Test- This test measures the levels of the neurotransmitters: dopamine, norepinephrine and epinephrine. Test for catecholamines measures the level of catecholamines in the plasma portion of blood. This test typically used to diagnose and/or monitor pheochromocytoma or neuroblastoma.

Cortisol Blood Lab– Your body's natural cortisol levels should be the highest in the morning, according to your body's circadian rhythm. If your AM levels are low, it can indicate an adrenal issue. This test will measure the level of cortisol in your blood.

Aldosterone Blood Lab– Blood test which measures the amount of aldosterone (ALD) in your blood. Physicians usually test your levels of renin and aldosterone simultaneously. (Also known as a plasma renin activity test or an aldosterone-renin ratio)

DHEA Blood Lab– Test which measures the blood level of dehydroepiandrosterone (DHEA) and dehydroepiandrosterone sulfate (DHEA-S).

Saliva Cortisol Test– Test which measures plasma free cortisol concentration in human saliva.

Urine Cortisol Test– Also called a urinary free cortisol (UFC) test. This test measures the total amount of cortisol excreted into urine over 24 hours.

It is important to appropriately evaluate the results of blood, saliva and urine cortisol testing. There is a difference between bound cortisol and free cortisol within the body. Testing metabolized cortisol evaluates how much cortisol is being created and cleared through the liver. Testing free cortisol evaluates how much cortisol is free to bind to receptors and allows for assessment of the circadian rhythm. The largest amount of cortisol in the body is bound to cortisol-binding globulin (CBG) and albumin. On average, less than 5% of circulating cortisol is unbound (free). Only unbound (free) cortisol can access the transporters in tissues that regulate metabolic and excretory clearance. Free cortisol is the biologically active cortisol. A small part of cortisol in the body is free. This amount of cortisol is vital, but levels of metabolized cortisol are the best evaluation of overall production of cortisol. Measuring both free and bound cortisol may provide a vital insight into the amount of cortisol metabolism and production. A total cortisol blood test measures both bound and free cortisol levels in the blood.

Standard Cortisol Ranges[5]

A normal adult range for cortisol levels in urine is between **3.5 and 45 micrograms per 24 hours**.

Reference ranges for salivary cortisol assay: **<0.4–3.6 nmol/L at 2300 h & 4.7–32.0 nmol/L at 0700 h.**

---

[5] Mayo Clinic. Cortisol, Free and Total, Serum.
https://www.mayocliniclabs.com/test-catalog/Clinical+and+Interpretive/65484

Standard 8 a.m. range for blood serum cortisol is between **6 and 23 micrograms per deciliter (mcg/dL)**

Additional Testing

Comprehensive Metabolic Panel (CMP)
The CMP test includes:
• Liver function (ALP, ALT, AST, Bilirubin)
• Kidney function (BUN, Creatinine)
• Electrolytes and fluid balance (Sodium, Potassium, Carbon Dioxide, Chloride)
• Proteins (Albumin, Total Protein)
• Blood sugar (Glucose)
• Calcium

CMP testing is helpful in evaluating adrenal disease patients because electrolyte imbalance can accompany adrenal insufficiency. The test also helps evaluate organ function, electrolytes, blood sugar, and blood proteins. Specifically, primary Addison's disease patients need to be aware of their potassium levels. Additionally, it is recommended that salt wasting forms of adrenal insufficiency have electrolytes evaluated and may require sodium supplementation or an adjustment in their fludrocortisone dosing to keep levels in a normal range.

Pre-Pump Planning

Before you begin the process of cortisol pumping, it is important to assess your life, health and disease management. The cortisol pump is not a cure for adrenal insufficiency and is not a treatment that is right for everyone. If you are well managed on the steroid replacement pills, the adrenal pump is excess money and effort you may not need. The pump is not an easy thing to acquire and the fight to get one takes a great deal of trouble, mental stamina and resources. **Research, learn and educate for yourself.**

Information you need to know:

What is your diagnosis?

What form of adrenal insufficiency do you have?

What is your quality of life?

Are you able to work, drive, do housework or function normally?

What have you tried to manage your adrenal disease?

What is your current daily dose of replacement steroid?

How much are you stress dosing?

What other medical issues do you have?

Are you able to afford the supplies and medication needed for the pump?

Insurance may or may not cover your pump, supplies or solu-cortef.

Steroid Options

Before starting the pump, it is important to explore all possible options to manage adrenal disease. Finding the right steroid is dependent on each adrenal insufficient patient. Variables like personal cortisol clearance rates, pain levels, health comorbidities, weight, stress management and physical activity will impact dosing needs. It is important to work with a physician who is proficient in managing adrenal disease to determine the most optimal steroid replacement medication.

Standard Treatments for Adrenal Insufficiency

The following list are the oral medications commonly prescribed for Adrenal Insufficiency.

This is not an all-inclusive list and not to be used to diagnose or replace medical care.

Cortisone Acetate- The acetate salt form of cortisone, a synthetic or semisynthetic analog of the naturally occurring cortisone hormone. Cortisone itself is inactive; it is converted in the liver to the active metabolite hydrocortisone.

Dexamethasone (Decadron)- Medication is used in the treatment of cancers such as leukemias, and lymphomas and to treat diseases involving destruction by the body's own immune system. Also used to treat adrenal insufficiency. Dexamethasone is a long-acting steroid and remains in blood circulation for approximately 16 hours after administration, with a half-life of about 4 hours.

Fludrocortisone (Florinef) – Synthetic medication used to treat salt wasting diseases such as primary Addison's disease. Fludrocortisone cannot be converted to another corticosteroid on the basis of anti-inflammatory potency. It is not a replacement for cortisol but is used in addition to cortisol replacement in some forms of adrenal disease.

Hydrocortisone (Cortef) - Medication is the most bio-identical form of cortisol. It is a short acting steroid used to treat autoimmune diseases, allergic reactions and also adrenal insufficiency. The pharmaceutical properties of the dosage of hydrocortisone are determined by intestinal absorption rate and the plasma concentration-time profile of hydrocortisone (cortisol) in a specific patient's body. There are many factors that cause or result in pharmacokinetic variability; therefore, the short elimination half-life of hydrocortisone is approximately 1.5 hours when given in traditional immediate-release dosage forms.

Methylprednisolone (Medrol)- Medication which is a synthetic corticosteroid and is mainly used to achieve prompt suppression of inflammation but can also be used to treat adrenal insufficiency.

Prednisolone (Prelone)- Synthetic glucocorticoid replacement medication used to treat adrenal insufficiency and also used to treat autoimmune diseases and allergic reactions.

Prednisone- Synthetic corticosteroid which mimics the action of cortisol produced in the body by the adrenal glands. Most often used for its potent anti-inflammatory effects, particularly in autoimmune and inflammatory diseases and conditions. Also used to treat adrenal insufficiency. Prednisone is inactive in the body and in order to be effective first must be converted to prednisolone by enzymes in the liver. Prednisone may not work as effectively in people with liver disease whose ability to convert prednisone to prednisolone is impaired.

Rayos- Long-acting corticosteroid medication in the form of delayed-release prednisone. This medication releases the action of prednisone about 4 hours after tablets are ingested. Used the treatment of such rheumatoid arthritis polymyalgia rheumatica and also adrenal insufficiency.

Steroid Equivalent Dose Conversion

20mg Hydrocortisone	0.8mg Dexamethasone	5mg Prednisone
5mg Prednisolone	5mg Cortisone	4mg MethylPrednisolone

Additional Care Protocols

DHEA Supplementation: (Dehydroepiandrosterone) and DHEA sulfate (DHEAS) are the major circulating adrenal steroids and substrates for peripheral sex hormone biosynthesis. In patients with adrenal insufficiency, glucocorticoid and mineralocorticoid deficiencies require lifelong replacement, but the associated near-total failure of DHEA synthesis is not typically corrected in current endocrine care protocols. However, research[6] shows that DHEA supplementation may increase quality of life in patients with adrenal insufficiency. Be sure to check with your physician before starting DHEA because there are risks. DHEA can raise the level of both male and female hormones, therefore supplementation can have a negative effect on certain types of hormone-sensitive cancers. Patients should also be aware that DHEA supplementation can worsen psychiatric conditions and may increase the risks of manic episodes.[7]

There are two forms of DHEA supplementation: DHEA and 7 Keto DHEA. 7 Keto DHEA is the preferred supplement because unlike DHEA, 7-keto-DHEA is not converted to steroid hormones such as androgen and estrogen.[8]

---

[6] Gurnell, E., Hunt, P., Curran, S., Conway, C., Pullenayegum, E., Huppert, F., . . . Chatterjee, V. (2008, February). Long-term dhea replacement in primary adrenal insufficiency: A randomized, controlled trial.

[7] Mayo Clinic (2021, February 12). DHEA. Retrieved from https://www.mayoclinic.org/drugs-supplements-dhea/art-20364199

[8] Behavorial Pharmacology. Author manuscript; available in PMC 2013 Jun 1.Published in final edited form as: Behav Pharmacol. 2012 Jun; 23(3): 250–261. doi: 10.1097/FBP.0b013e32835342d2

Sodium Chloride Tablets

In salt wasting forms of adrenal insufficiency, patients may find benefit from sodium chloride tablets and can be safely used as an electrolyte replenisher.

Intravenous Infusions

Patients with severe forms of adrenal insufficiency often struggle with hydration[9], electrolyte homeostasis, heart rate and blood pressure dysregulation and may find benefit from infusion solutions such as saline and/or lactated ringers. Patients with primary adrenal insufficiency (Addison's disease) need to use caution with lactated ringers because they contain potassium, which can be abnormal in the cases of primary Addison's.

Hydrocortisone Injections

Patients who have not stabilized on oral cortisol steroid replacement may find benefit from switching to injections of hydrocortisone. Some adrenal patients find this is an effective transitional method to try if they are not stable on traditional oral steroids and are in the process to begin the cortisol pumping method. Hydrocortisone injections can be given in 1mg increments and doses can be tailored more specifically than oral corticosteroids.

---

[9] *The Journal of Clinical Endocrinology & Metabolism*, Volume 94, Issue 4, 1 April 2009, Pages 1059–1067, https://doi.org/10.1210/jc.2009-0032

Supplies needed:

- Solu-Cortef 100mg vials
- Saline or Bacteriostatic Water
- Skin Prep such as alcohol swabs
- 3ML Syringes to reconstitute Solu-Cortef
- Syringes or "insulin" needles for injections

Instructions:

Each 100mg vial of Solu-Cortef will need to be reconstituted with 1mL of saline or bacteriostatic water for a 1:1 ratio. (1mg=1unit) Injections should be administered in the layer of fat just below the skin in abdomen, upper arms, thighs or buttocks. Patients should rotate injection sites. Physicians need to calculate a baseline cortisol dose and also create a dosing schedule based on circadian rhythm protocols, the patient's cortisol clearance, activity level and health comorbidities. For example, if a patient was taking 40mg of hydrocortisone tablets, that would equate to 40units of solucortef to be administered in the form of multiple daily injections.

Lab Work

To best manage adrenal insufficiency, it is helpful to determine an adrenal patient's cortisol clearance rate. The most common way to assess this is by a "day curve" test, where a patient's blood serum cortisol levels are drawn every hour for twenty-four hours.

This test is difficult to obtain, alternative testing can be performed. Many laborites have a multi-specimen lab tests for cortisol.

Multi Specimen Lab Test available in the U.S:

Quest Lab- Cortisol, Six specimens (Test Code 6734. CPT Code 82533 (x6)

Labcorp- Cortisol, Six specimens (Test code: 024091. CPT Code: 82533(x6)

Ideally, one would want a 24-hour cortisol panel completed, but since a day curve may be difficult to obtain the previously mentioned tests will still give an insight into the cortisol clearance rates of an adrenal insufficient patient on cortisol replacement medications. This information will help an endocrinologist or other physician to calculate a basal cortisol distribution dose.

It is important to note that the cortisol pump is only as effective as the information programmed into it, which is why proper evaluation and testing is necessary for the effectiveness of this treatment. As previously mentioned, there are many factors which will determine an adrenal insufficient patient's cortisol needs.

Cortisol testing is vital to the success of the cortisol pumping method. It is important to evaluate how quickly an adrenal insufficient person's body sustains cortisol in their system. Rates need to be calculated to how fast a person's body metabolizes cortisol in addition to circadian rhythm percentages and empirical evidence of low cortisol symptoms and quality of life.

Chapter 3: Starting the Cortisol Pumping Process

Finding a Pump Friendly Physician

The first step to cortisol pumping is establishing a care plan with a licensed medical professional. This can be a difficult challenge when trying to find a physician to manage your care with the pumping method, as most have never heard of it. It may take you many tries to find a physician willing to manage your care with the cortisol pumping method.

Send your research, your health information, everything you can to the physician before your appointment, so they are aware of your intentions beforehand. It may benefit you to write a letter to the endocrinologist prior to your appointment that explains your diagnosis, failed treatments and desire to be on the pump. They may or may not be receptive to your request and alerting them of your intentions beforehand may save you time, money and effort. You can find an example of a "pump proposal" letter and cortisol pumping research in the resources chapter of this book.

Keep in mind this treatment is a nuance and the doctor may or may not be receptive to your request. You may have to query multiple physicians before you find one who is willing to manage your care on the pump.

Choosing a Pump System

There are multiple different pump systems available. Determining what infusion pump company works best for you will depend on your personal cortisol needs, what your insurance will cover, your lifestyle and your location.

Though the concept of all pumps are basically the same, some have different features such as being waterproof or tubeless.

Choosing a pump system is a decision you and your overseeing physician can make based on insurance coverage, activity level and accessibility.

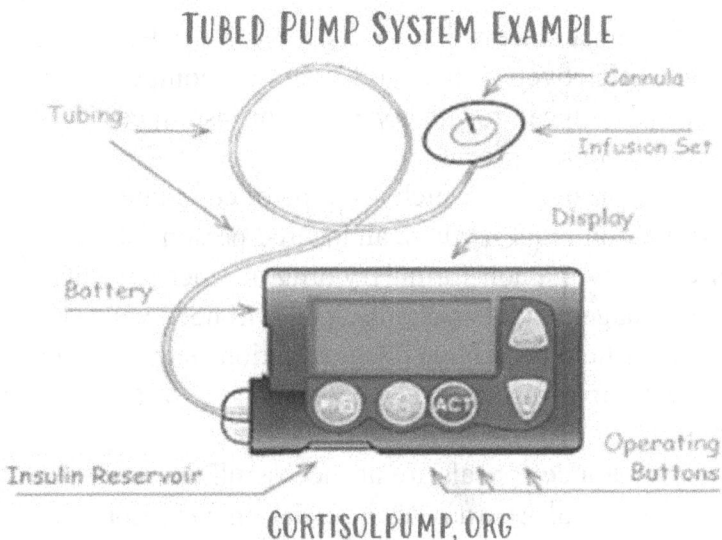

TUBED PUMP SYSTEM EXAMPLE

Tubing

Cannula

Infusion Set

Display

Battery

Operating Buttons

Insulin Reservoir

CORTISOLPUMP, ORG

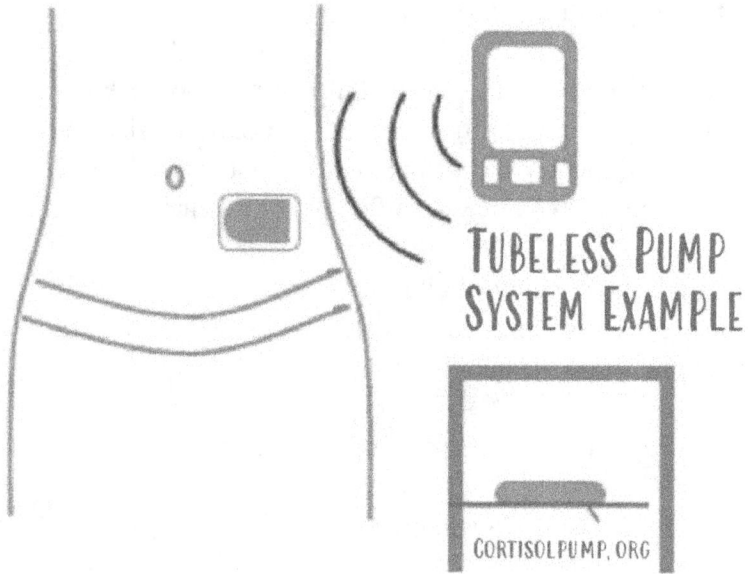

TUBELESS PUMP
SYSTEM EXAMPLE

CORTISOLPUMP.ORG

Obtaining Insurance Approval

What your insurance will cover is completely dependent on your specific coverage plan and insurance company. If you are denied, you can file an appeal. Your insurance company's appeal process may require you to file a formulary exemption, which is a type of coverage determination request where an insured person asks the insurer to cover a non-formulary drug or amend the plan's usage management restrictions. You will need your physician's help to provide documentation as to why the non-formulary drug should be covered.

If your insurance appeals are unsuccessful, there are other options. Adrenal Alternatives Foundation has resources to help adrenal patients acquire pumps in a safe and legal manner, with or without insurance coverage.

It is also an option to cash purchase pumps and supplies specifically from companies if you have a prescription from your overseeing physician.

Chapter 4: Creating a Care Plan

You will need your overseeing physician to write prescriptions for Solu-Cortef vials, the infusion pump and supplies needed to manage your care on the cortisol pumping method.

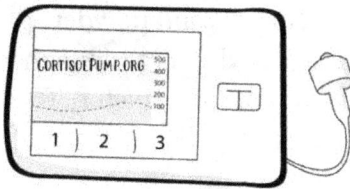

CORTISOL PUMP SUPPLIES NEEDED:
ALCOHOL PREP PADS
INFUSION PUMP
INFUSION SET / RESERVOIRS
SALINE OR BACTERIOSTATIC WATER
SOLU-CORTEF
SYRINGES

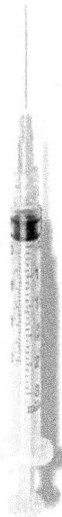

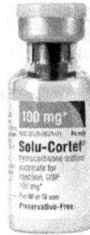

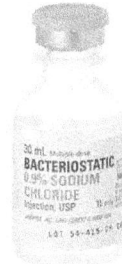

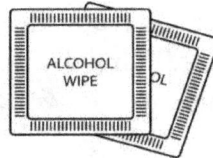

Prescriptions & Items Needed:
- Alcohol Prep Pads
- Infusion Pump
- Infusion Sets & Reservoirs
- Saline or Bacteriostatic Water
- Solu-Cortef
- Syringes

Additionally helpful supplies:

- Band-Aids
- Hibiclens solution
- Medical paper tape
- Skin Tac
- Tegaderms
- Label stating your pump contains cortisol and not insulin
- Sharps Container

Choosing a Solu-Cortef Ratio

Solu-Cortef comes in two forms, actovials and powder vials. The actovials are Solu-Cortef powder that is attached with 2ML of saline solution at the top of the canister. The powder vials are only Solu-Cortef.

With actovials, the ratio is 2:1. This means that 2ml of solution is equal to 2mg of cortisol because 100mg of solu-cortef was mixed with the 2ml of saline contained in the canister and reconstituted before adding it into the pump reservoir. Pump distribution rates will be calculated according to this.

Example-If a patient takes 20 mg daily their basal rate will be 40units.

2units= 2mg at the 2:1 ratio.

With the powder solu-cortef vials, patients can run a 1:1 ratio by mixing the 100mg of Solu-Cortef powder with

1ML of saline or bacteriostatic water and reconstituting it with a syringe before adding it into the pump reservoir.

Example-If a patient takes 35 mg daily, their basal rate will be 35units.

1unit= 1mg at the 1:1 ratio.

With the 1:1 ratio, less volume will be pushed through an infusion site and math calculations on bolusing and rate increases are simpler.

Setting Basal Rates

Rates need to be calculated according to the results of the cortisol clearance testing, circadian rhythm percentages, empirical patient symptoms and overall wellness. The body naturally produces cortisol at different intervals throughout the day, the highest being in the morning to generate the natural waking response and the lowest in the evening to induce sleep. Cortisol levels will also rise in accordance to stressors such as exercise, pain or emotional situations. All these factors must be considered when programming an infusion pump for cortisol distribution.

Patients need to work with their physicians to calculate the best possible care plan for quality of life. It is vital to keep track of blood pressure, heart rate, overall feeling of wellness, low cortisol symptoms, stress tolerance, energy levels and physical stamina. Every adrenal patient is different and steroid replacement needs to be tailored to each patient depending on their health status and lifestyle. Steroids can cause side effects and the right dosing at the right time is imperative to achieve quality of life. Steroid dosing may differ from day to day depending on the body's physical cortisol needs, which can change in times of stressors such as injury, surgery, pain, emotional situations or grief. Replacement needs may differ from day to day depending on the stressors the body may be exposed to. It is important to work with your overseeing physician to establish a basal dose and proper rate distribution.

Cortisol replacement therapy needs to be a personalized, calculated process where the following factors are considered.

1– **Your personal absorption**. Clearance testing labs can be done to determine how quickly your body metabolizes cortisol.

2– **Your daily basal dose needs**. Every adrenal patient is different. Your dose will depend on your specific body's needs according to your health status, comorbidities, pain levels, weight, and cortisol clearance.

3– **Your distribution rates/times**. Cortisol replacement needs to be administered as closely to the circadian rhythm as possible. 24-hour profiles can be programmed to match the body's natural cortisol production.

Physicians can evaluate rates with the 24-hour cortisol day curve testing to evaluate the efficacy of the cortisol replacement after a patient begins the infusion pumping method. However, it must be understood that quality of life should be the standard to which the efficacy of the cortisol pumping method is judged. If a patient is still suffering with low cortisol symptoms, the pump rates should be re-evaluated despite lab work being within a normal range.

Circadian rhythm dosing[10] is essential to effective cortisol replacement. Cortisol regulates the body's internal processes that regulate the sleep-wake cycle. Circadian rhythm refers to the physical, mental, and behavioral patterns that follow a daily cycle in human life. Cortisol is deeply crucial to circadian rhythm modulation. Oral hydrocortisone replacement cannot reproduce this physiological rhythm, therefore adrenal insufficient patients may be inadvertently are under or over replaced within the same 24-hour dosing period. This suggests why a majority of patients diagnosed with adrenal insufficiency suffer from a poor quality of life, with increased mortality rates, sleep disturbances, impaired psychological wellness. Cortisol replication needs to be administered according to circadian rhythm protocols; the highest cortisol would be produced by the body in the morning and levels slowly decrease throughout the day to allow for sleep at night. The body requires cortisol 24/7, however it needs higher levels in the early morning to induce the body's cortisol waking response.[11]

[10] Chan, Sharon, and Miguel Debono. "Replication of Cortisol Circadian Rhythm: New Advances in Hydrocortisone Replacement Therapy." Therapeutic Advances in Endocrinology and Metabolism. SAGE Publications, June 2010. Web.

[11] Endocrine Reviews, Volume 38, Issue 1, 1 February 2017, Pages 3–45, https://doi.org/10.1210/er.2015-1080 Published: 17 October 2016

Cortisol Secretion Percentages over a 24-hour period[12]:

6:00am to noon 35% of cortisol is produced.

Noon to 6:00pm 20% of cortisol is produced.

6:00pm to Midnight 15% of cortisol is produced.

Midnight to 6:00am 30% of cortisol is produced.

Updosing and Sick Rates

What is updosing?

The pump truly puts adrenal patients in control of their cortisol distribution in a way that steroid pills cannot. In situations of physical or emotional stress where "updosing" is needed, the pump can immediately administer a bolus, which is extra cortisol administered through the pump canula at the amount you select. Instead of having to wait 30-90 minutes for pills to metabolize, the cortisol can be absorbed faster and may be able to better help prevent an adrenal crisis.

It is not only important to establish a basal rate but also to create a plan for updosing or bolusing for times when extra cortisol is needed. The amount of extra cortisol needed will depend on personal cortisol clearance and the body's stress tolerance. Adrenal patients may exhibit low cortisol in various symptoms. It is vital to know your own personal signs and symptoms of low cortisol and updose at the first symptom. Playing cortisol catch up is a dangerous game that no adrenal patient needs to play. It is imperative that

---

[12] Hindmarsh, P.,CAHISUS, Circadian Rhythm Dosing. Retrieved from www.cahisus.co.uk/pdf/CIRCADIAN%20RHYTHM%20DOSING.pdf

adrenal insufficient patients updose at the first sign of low cortisol to prevent an adrenal crisis and always carry an emergency cortisol injection.

What are sick rates?

Sick rates are delivery rates set to administer elevated amounts of medication to manage sickness, injury or stress which require more medication such as insulin or solucortef.

It is important to note that double doses of cortisol do not double the blood levels[13]. In times of sickness, infection and recovery a basal sick rate may be needed. Sick rates are not set according to circadian rhythm and provide a flatter dosing distribution of cortisol.

Bolusing/Updosing Protocols:

- Exercise
- Emotional Stress (Grief, Trauma, etc.)
- Physical Exertion (Household tasks, etc.)
- Emergency Situations (Accidents, etc.)
- Surgery
- Sickness (Fever, Vomiting, etc.)
- Pain
- Extreme Temperatures (Heat or Cold)

Sites and Absorption Factors

Parts of your body where subcutaneous fat is are optimal sites for the absorption of Solu-Cortef, insulin and other absorbable medications. Recommended site placements are: the abdomen, back of arms, thighs, and upper buttocks.

---

[13] Hindmarsh, P., 2017. *Congenital Adrenal Hyperplasia*. Elsvier Academic Press, p.384.

Issues such as scar tissue and surgical adhesions can impact a person's ability to absorb their medication. Absorption rate fluctuations can vary from one person to the other. Sites should never be severely painful or exhibit blood. If they do, remove the site and put in a new one. If you sense your cortisol levels are dropping, change the site immediately. **"If in doubt, change it out"** has become a mantra amongst adrenal pumpers. As previously mentioned, playing "cortisol catch up" is a life-threatening game of misery that no adrenal patient needs to play.

The frequency of when sites must be changed is dependent on the specific pumping system you choose. Some infusion sites can stay in the body for up to three days.

Absorption rates may be less effective the longer a site is in the body, especially if high volumes of medication are being administered through the cannula into the tissue.

If a bolus is administered and it is not effectively treating low cortisol symptoms, it is recommended to change the site. The longer an adrenal patient goes without adequate cortisol replacement, the more difficult it will be to stabilize them.

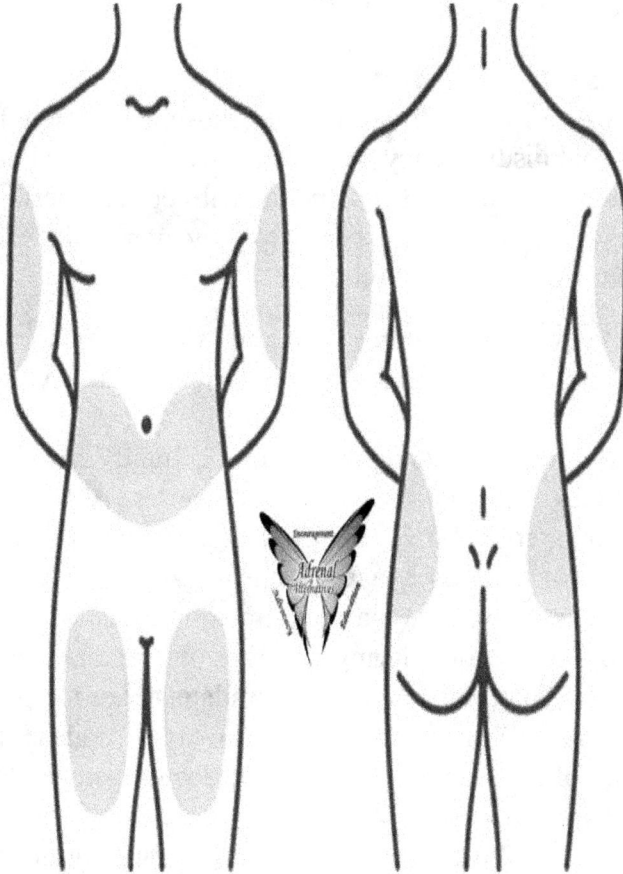

Infusion Site Locations for Cortisol Pumping

For more information on the cortisol pumping method visit
Adrenal Alternatives Foundation at adrenalalternatives.com

Chapter 5: Life with the Pump

Exercise

Exercise can be a difficult task for those with severe forms of adrenal insufficiency. Any extra stressor on the body can be potentially deadly for someone with cortisol deficiency. However, exercise is necessary to prevent muscle wasting and physical deterioration.

Discuss exercise concerns with a physician. You can have a physical evaluation done to assess how receptive your body is to exercise. Once you are physically cleared, you can also try low impact and safe options to lightly introduce your body to more activity. Find an exercise regimen that does not overwhelm your body. It is also important to give your body the cortisol that it needs to handle the extra physical activity. This may require an increase in your cortisol dose before, during or after your exercise session. Talk with your physician and formulate a plan for updosing for exercise. With the pump, you can bolus (updose) the number of milligrams you and your doctor have decided on before you exercise. You can also set elevated rates to be administered during and after your workout routine by setting a temp basal increase.

Electrolyte balance and hydration are also extremely important when exercising with adrenal insufficiency. Hyponatremia and hyperkalemia are two major electrolyte abnormalities that can occur in adrenal insufficiency. Hyponatremia is mediated by increased release of antidiuretic hormone (ADH) which results in water retention and a reduction in the plasma sodium concentration. ADH levels increase when plasma cortisol levels are low, therefore making it beneficial to updose before physical activity to prevent low cortisol.[14]

It is much harder to elevate your cortisol levels once they hit a low point, so it is recommended that you bolus or set elevated rates before you begin your workout. Talk with your physician to form a plan on cortisol updosing before you begin an exercise regimen. Be sure that you always wear a medical alert bracelet that states you are cortisol dependent and you carry an emergency injection with you. If you work out at a gym, you may want to provide the staff with an emergency injection instruction handout.

---

[14]Tafuri, K., Dr., & Bowden, S. A., Dr. (2020, December 03). What is the role of electrolyte level measurement in the workup of pediatric adrenal insufficiency (Addison disease)?

Neary N, Nieman L. Adrenal insufficiency: etiology, diagnosis, and treatment. Curr Opin Endocrinol Diabetes Obes. 2010 Apr 6. [Medline].

Emergency Cortisol Injection Instructions

1–Remove the two-chamber vial containing SoluCortef ActOVial from the packaging box.

2–Press the colored cap down to mix solvent with the powder solution of hydrocortisone.

3–Mix the contents until the powder is completely dissolved. The powder solution of hydrocortisone is completely dissolved once the solution is clear.

4–Remove the protective disc from the center of the plastic cap of the SoluCortef vial.

5–Wipe top of vial with alcohol swab to sterilize before inserting syringe into vial.

6–Insert the syringe into the vial. Turn the vial upside down and draw the entire solution into the syringe.

7–Clean the adrenal patient's skin with an alcohol skin prep where you intend on injecting the needle.

8–Hold the syringe like a dart, and push the needle for 2/3 of its length into the chosen injection site at a right angle to the skin. Give injection into intramuscular tissue sites such as the buttock, upper arm or in the upper thigh muscle.

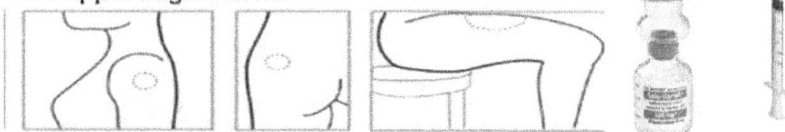

Always administer an emergency cortisol injection **immediately** at the first sign of an adrenal crisis, which will result in death if left untreated.

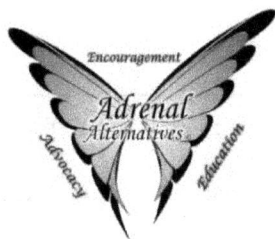

For more information visit adrenalalternatives.com

Showering

If you have a non-waterproof tubed system, you will need to pause your cortisol distribution and disconnect from your pump to shower. You can also plan your shower days around your site changes or simply disconnect from the pump and cover your site with a tegaderm and reconnect after your shower. If you have a tubed waterproof pump however, you can shower with it by using a waist or arm band to keep it in place. There are also completely waterproof and tubeless pumps where showering is completely uninhibited.

Traveling

Traveling with the pump through airports, train or bus stations is much easier with preparation and documentation. It is a good idea to have documentation written from your doctor of your diagnosis, what to do for emergency protocols and the necessity of your pump. Most travel companies and airlines will allow you to call ahead and request disability services and you may even can have baggage fees waived if your luggage contains medical equipment. Be sure you are traveling with proper documentation and your supplies are organized. Always have more than enough supplies for the length of your stay and label everything with your name, diagnosis and treatment protocols. Planning ahead can make a major difference in the ease and success of your travels with the cortisol pump. You may also want to consider bringing a backup pump or subcutaneous injection supplies in case your pump fails during your travels. It is not recommended that certain pumps go through the machines at the airport, so you can request a hand check with TSA instead. Not all pumps need this precaution. Be sure to research the specifics of the pump system you are traveling with.

Intimacy

Intimacy should not be inhibited by pump use, but patients and their partners should use caution to ensure sites are not pulled out of the skin or damaged. Research[15] findings have shown that cortisol has many implications for both reproductive health and sexual function, which suggests that you may need to updose before you engage in sexual activity. Any excess stress on the body may require additional cortisol replacement, even good stress. Talk with your physician about forming a plan to updose if you feel low cortisol symptoms during or after sexual activity.

Surgery Protocols

During a surgical procedure, the body will require an increase in steroid dosing. Surgery is one of the most prominent activators of the HPA axis. Researchers[1] have reported HPA axis function during and after surgical procedures that plasma cortisol levels increase significantly. In patients without the presence of adrenal insufficiency, cortisol production rates increased to 75-150 mg/day after major surgery. This is one reason why the cortisol pump is such a benefit for adrenal insufficient patients because the pumping method provides continuous infusion even during medical procedures. A person can then receive continuous cortisol just like a non-adrenal

---

[15] J Sex Med. Author manuscript; available in PMC 2009 Jun 30. Published in final edited form as:
J Sex Med. 2008 Sep; 5(9): 2111–2118.
Published online 2008 Jul 4. doi: 10.1111/j.1743-6109.2008.00922.x

insufficiency person's body would naturally do. In adrenal insufficient patients, the recommendations on increased cortisol coverage differs depending on the length and severity of the procedure being performed. It is important to note that adrenal insufficiency patients will always require additional glucocorticoid supplementation during surgery, but there is no uniform standard accepted regimen for glucocorticoid replacement therapy. It is the best clinical practice to treat the patient instead of following a textbook. If a patient with adrenal insufficiency is declining, the administration of more cortisol should be a first line treatment protocol.

However, there are suggested recommendations: [2]

For Minor Surgery: Double or triple the usual daily dose of glucocorticoid until recovery. Intravenous hydrocortisone 25 mg or equivalent at start of procedure. Usual replacement dose after procedure.

For Dental Procedures: Under local anesthesia, double the daily dose of glucocorticoid on day of procedure. Inject 100mg emergency cortisol injection if patient presents with adrenal crisis symptoms.

For Moderate Surgery: Intravenous hydrocortisone 75 mg/day on day of procedure (25 mg 8-hourly). Intravenous hydrocortisone 25 mg 8-hourly until recovery. Taper over next 1–2 days to usual replacement dose in uncomplicated cases.

For Major Surgery:
Intravenous hydrocortisone 150 mg/day (50 mg 8-hourly)
Taper over next 2–3 days only once clinical condition
stabilizes.

For critical illness/intensive care/major trauma or life-threatening complications:
200 mg/day intravenous hydrocortisone (50 mg 6-hourly,
or by continuous infusion)

Note: There is no universally agreed upon standard dose or
duration of exogenous steroids used to treat adrenal
insufficiency. Clinicians must be observant of a patient's
vital signs, empirical evidence and quality of life. It is also
imperative clinicians be aware of the symptoms of adrenal
crisis, which can widely vary in patients. In the event these
symptoms should arise, an immediate dose of
glucocorticoids should be administered until patient
stabilizes.

Cautions:
Before your surgery, be sure that your healthcare team is
aware of your use of the cortisol pump. Ensure your pump
is labeled that it is cortisol and not insulin and it is
documented that the pump should remain attached to you
prior to, during and after your procedure. If possible, speak
with the anesthesiologist and surgeon beforehand and
inform them of the previously mentioned concerns.

[1]

Management of adrenal insufficiency during the stress of medical
illness and surgery: Jung, C. and Inder, W. (2008). [online]
Australasian Medical Publishing Company.

[2] Perioperative Steroid Management: Approaches Based on Current Evidence: Collard MD, C., Saatee, M.D, S., Reidy, M.D, A. and Liu, M.D, M. (2017). [online] Anesthesiology: Trusted Evidence Discovery in Practice.

Chapter 6: Resources

Appeal Letters

This is an example of an insurance appeal letter you and your doctor can use to contest your insurance's decision should they deny the pump or supply coverage. This letter was created by the Adrenal Alternatives Foundation for use in the United States to achieve coverage for the supplies needed to manage the cortisol pumping method. Individual results may vary on approval status depending on your specific plan's coverage.

Example Insurance Appeal Letter:

Address to insurance company or appeal source
Date
Appeal Regarding-*Name of denied pump*
Add your plan information such as
Formulary ID
Plan Type
Enrollee ID number
Contract ID
Plan ID
Group Number
Your Name and DOB
Policy Holder and DOB (omit if you are the policy holder)
Appeal for coverage of denied RX for pump

Name
Diagnosis
DOB
Applicable ICD-10 Diagnosis Codes (Suggestions-
Adrenal Insufficiency (Addison's Disease) E27.1
Management of infusion pump Z45.1

NAME OF PUMP is FDA approved for chronic drug administration. The NAME OF PUMP meets the recommendations for chronic glucocorticoid administration to treat Adrenal Insufficiency. Adrenal insufficiency is the failure of the body to produce cortisol, which is a life sustaining hormone. For comparison, it is similar to the disease of Type 1 diabetes, which renders a person insulin deficient. Adrenal insufficiency renders a person cortisol deficient, and cortisol replacement is necessary to sustain life. Administration of corticosteroids is the only treatment for adrenal insufficiency. PATIENT NAME requires this treatment and as their physician, I have prescribed NAME OF PUMP as the recommended clinical treatment that is necessary to sustain their life. According to the Department of Health and Human Services Centers for Medicare and Medicaid Services Medicare Coverage Issues Manual Section 60-14 A:"6. Other uses of external infusion pumps are covered if the contractor's medical staff verifies the appropriateness of the therapy and of the prescribed pump for the individual patient." According to above stated criteria, patient meets criteria for coverage. According to Khalil A, Ahmed F, Alzohaili O. Continuous glucocorticoid infusion for adrenal insufficiency is a novel approach to deliver corticosteroids in patients with poor cortisol absorption. Presented at: American Association of Clinical Endocrinologists 28th Annual Scientific & Clinical Congress; April 24-28, 2019; Los Angeles, CA. "The results indicated that the use of cortisol pumps was associated with a 78.5% risk reduction for adrenal crisis compared with oral corticosteroids, in addition to reducing the number of adrenal crises, this method was found to be associated with better symptom control and quality of life. Continuous pulsatile cortisol replacement via pump is an option for management of severe adrenal insufficiency in patients unresponsive to oral therapy."

According to the Right to Try Act, this patient should have access to this treatment. (a) IN GENERAL.—Chapter V of the Federal Food, Drug, and Cosmetic Act is amended by inserting after section 561A (21 U.S.C. 360bbb–0) the following: "SEC. 561B.INVESTIGATION "SEC. 561B. INVESTIGATIONAL DRUGS FOR USE BY ELIGIBLE PATIENTS. "(a) DEFINITIONS.—For purposes of this section— "(1) the term 'eligible patient' means a patient— "(A) who has been diagnosed with a life-threatening disease or condition (as defined in section 312.81 of title 21, Code of Federal Regulations (or any successor regulations)); "(B) who has exhausted approved treatment options and is unable to participate in a clinical trial involving the eligible investigational drug, as certified by a physician, who— "(i) is in good standing with the physician's licensing organization or board; and "(ii) will not be compensated directly by the manufacturer for so certifying; and "(C) who has provided to the treating physician written informed consent regarding the eligible investigational drug, or, as applicable, on whose behalf a legally authorized representative of the patient has provided such consent.

PATIENT NAME has been diagnosed with adrenal insufficiency and cannot sustain life without administration of glucocorticoid medication. Patient has not responded to oral corticosteroid and therefore, the denied treatment NAME OF PUMP is vital and life sustaining for this patient, as there is no alternative treatment for glucocorticoid administration in the management of adrenal insufficiency. According to medically indicated criteria, patient meets criteria for coverage and denying this prescription would not only be inhumane but also lead to imminent death for this patient.

Physician Signature

_____

Example Pump Proposal Letter:

Date
Name of Medical Practice
Address

Dear Dr.'s Name,
I am writing this letter in preparation for my appointment with you on DATE OF APPOINTMENT. I am a new patient to your practice and wanted to explain my history and objective beforehand in order to achieve the most beneficial results possible. I'm confident that with your experience and credentials you will be able to help me manage my care. I have been diagnosed with DIAGNOSIS. I am seeking a physician willing to help manage my adrenal disease with the cortisol pump. This treatment uses the concept of an insulin pump, but instead, it delivers Solu-cortef through the cannula instead of insulin. This allows adrenal insufficient patients like me to closely replicate the circadian rhythm in a way that taking oral tablets cannot, therefore improving quality of life and minimizing side effects. I am seeking a physician willing to manage me on this treatment. I currently take MEDICATION AND DOSE OF STEROID and struggle with HEALTH ISSUES. I believe the pump will improve my health and hope you will consider managing my care. I look forward to meeting you. Thank you for your time.

Sincerely,
YOUR NAME

Adrenal Alternatives Foundation Resources

Adrenal Alternatives Foundation is a 501c3 nonprofit patient advocacy organization dedicated to education, encouragement, and advocacy for all forms of adrenal disease. We have the following programs to help improve the lives of adrenal disease sufferers.

Cortisol Pump Advocacy
Oral steroid medications are the standard treatment to manage cortisol deficiency caused by adrenal insufficiency. The standard medication, hydrocortisone has a blood serum half-life of 90 minutes, which requires taking these tablets multiple times daily to replace cortisol. For patients who cannot absorb or metabolize oral steroids, adrenal insufficiency becomes a death sentence. But with an infusion pump, an adrenal insufficient patient can receive a constant supply of cortisol. Side effects due to malabsorption can be eliminated and patients have reported to have improved quality of life. This method is a lifesaving intervention for those who cannot absorb oral steroid medications. It has also been shown to lessen the prevalence of adrenal crises and hospitalizations due to low cortisol. This method is an off-label use of the infusion pump and there are very little resources to help patients achieve this life saving treatment. We are currently the only nonprofit organization in the world helping adrenal patients access this method. We are dedicated to providing adrenal insufficient patients who have failed traditional oral steroid treatment with the resources to safely and legally begin the cortisol pumping method. This involves educating physicians on how to manage this protocol and also ensuring patients have affordable access to a pump and

supplies. Our clinical team provides care plan guidelines to physicians seeking to manage the cortisol pumping method. Our team is dedicated to helping patients obtain insurance approval and we have aligned with the organization CR3 to create the Pumps for Purpose program where we provide pumps and supplies to adrenal patients, with or without insurance coverage.

Adrenal Awareness Initiative
Our Adrenal Awareness Initiative is a program our clinical team has created with downloadable materials such as: printable pamphlets, power point presentations, educational videos and advocacy images designed by our clinical team to educate patients, caregivers, family members, physicians, paramedics and all other medical professionals on how to recognize and manage adrenal insufficiency. These materials are available on our website and we also mail awareness packets with the complete program enclosed.

Publications
Adrenal Alternatives Foundation has published the book, Adrenal Insufficiency 101: A Patient's Guide to Managing Adrenal Insufficiency that contains factual information supported by credible medical sources, research and patient surveys on how to effectively manage adrenal insufficiency.

Legislative Work
We are actively working to change legislation that all qualified EMS personnel in the USA are authorized to administer the lifesaving Solu-Cortef injection, which is not

currently the case. Not all emergency medical personnel are allowed to administer lifesaving cortisol replacement medication and most ambulances do not have it on board. We are working to change this on a local, state and federal level. We have aligned with organizations such as Rare Disease Legislative Advocates, CIAAG- Chronic Illness Advocacy and Awareness Group, Danny's Dose and Adrenal Insufficiency Protocols who actively work to legislate for patient rights. Adrenal Alternatives Foundation also represents adrenal disease directly in congress through the Rare Disease Congressional Caucus. Our team proudly serves on the COVID19 response, Public Policy and Healthcare Access congressional committees. We are also active members of the Rare Disease Legislative Advocates Program and work alongside local, state and federal representatives to be a voice for the adrenal community.

Research
We are working to create technology to manage adrenal disease. Unlike diabetics, there is currently no meter to check cortisol blood levels. Adrenal patients must be constantly vigilant of their cortisol levels, which can drop in an instant. Research and technology advances are desperately needed, as the mortality rate of adrenal crisis remains high and quality of life is low for many patients diagnosed with adrenal insufficiency.

Resources
Downloadable Materials:
Subcutaneous Hydrocortisone Injection Protocols
Emergency Cortisol Injection Instructions
Cortisol Pump Proposal Letter to Your Doctor
How to Treat an Adrenal Crisis

How to be Tested for Adrenal Insufficiency
Guide to the Cortisol Pump
Guide to Steroids
Explaining Adrenal Disease
Cortisol Pump Insurance Appeal Letter
EMS/Paramedic Protocol Advocacy Instructions
Adrenal Disease- Testing, Treatments and Symptoms
Caregiver Guide to Adrenal Disease

Podcast Content
Steroids Save lives- The risks and benefits of steroid
replacement in adrenal insufficiency
Understanding Steroids Series with Dr. Megan
How to Manage Weight on Steroids
The Cortisol Pump- Everything you need to know
Interview with SOLUtion Medical- Creator of the Twistject
Cortisol Emergency Injector
Quality of Life Conversation Series
Townhall Meetings with Congressional Caucus Reps

Adrenal Alternatives Foundation is doing all we can to
improve and save lives through our previously mentioned
programs. The Adrenal Alternatives Foundation is
registered with the IRS as a 501(c)3 nonprofit organization
(EIN: 83-3629121)

For more information you can visit our social media:
Website: Adrenalalternatives.com
Instagram: AdrenalAlternativesFoundation
Facebook.com/hopeforadrenaldisease
Twitter: @AdrenalAdvocate
Podcast: anchor.fm/adrenal-alternatives-foundation
Youtube: Adrenal Alternatives Foundation Channel

Donations can be electronically accepted at
Paypal.me/adrenalalternatives

A comprehensive list of research supporting the cortisol
pump method can be found at:
adrenalalternatives.com/resources/

You can also find more information at cortisolpump.org

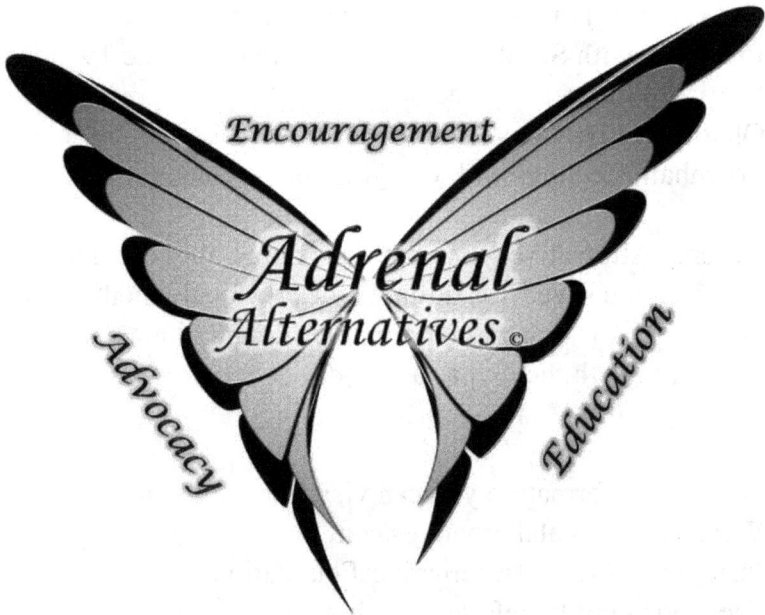

Sources:

Hindmarsh, P., 2017. Congenital Adrenal Hyperplasia. Elsvier Academic Press, p.384.

"Guidance Portal." U.S. Department of Health and Human Services Guidance Portal. 31 Dec. 2020. Web. 19 Feb. 2021. https://www.hhs.gov/guidance/document/medicare-coverage-issues-manual-transmittal-143>.

FDA. "Right to Try Act." U.S. Food and Drug Administration. 14 Jan. 2020. Web.

Elshimy, Ghada. "Adrenal Crisis." StatPearls [Internet]. U.S. National Library of Medicine, 20 Nov. 2020. Web.

"Diagnosing Adrenal Gland Disorders." Eunice Kennedy Shriver National Institute of Child Health and Human Development. U.S. Department of Health and Human Services, 31 Jan. 2017. Web. Available at: https://www.nichd.nih.gov/health/topics/adrenalgland/conditioninfo/diagnosed

Tafuri, K., Dr., & Bowden, S. A., Dr. (2020, December 03). What is the role of electrolyte level measurement in the workup of pediatric adrenal insufficiency (Addison disease)? medscape.com/answers/919077-167142/what-is-the-role-of-electrolyte-level-measurement-in-the-workup-of-pediatric-adrenal-insufficiency-addison-disease

Neary N, Nieman L. Adrenal insufficiency: etiology, diagnosis and treatment. Endocrinology, Diabetes & Obesity. 2010 Apr 6. [Medline]. https://pubmed.ncbi.nlm.nih.gov/20375886/

Mayo Clinic Laborites (n.d.). Cortisol, Free and Total, Serum. Retrieved from www.mayocliniclabs.com/test-catalog/Clinical+and+Interpretive/65484

Gurnell, E., Hunt, P., Curran, S., Conway, C., Pullenayegum, E., Huppert, F., . . . Chatterjee, V. (2008, February). Long-term dhea replacement in primary adrenal insufficiency: A randomized, controlled trial. Retrieved from www.ncbi.nlm.nih.gov/pmc/articles/PMC2729149/

Mayo Clinic (2021, February 12). DHEA. Retrieved from https://www.mayoclinic.org/drugs-supplements-dhea/art-20364199

Behavorial Pharmacology. Author manuscript; available in PMC 2013 Jun 1.Published in final edited form as: Behav Pharmacol. 2012 Jun; 23(3): 250–261. doi: 10.1097/FBP.0b013e32835342d2

Chan, Sharon, and Miguel Debono. "Replication of Cortisol Circadian Rhythm: New Advances in Hydrocortisone Replacement Therapy." Therapeutic Advances in Endocrinology and Metabolism. SAGE Publications, June 2010. Web. www.ncbi.nlm.nih.gov/pmc/articles/PMC3475279

Hindmarsh, P., & CAHISUS (n.d.). Circadian Rhythm Dosing. Retrieved from: www.cahisus.co.uk/pdf/CIRCADIAN%20RHYTHM%20DOSING.pdf

Endocrine Reviews, Volume 38, Issue 1, 1 February 2017, Pages 3–45, https://doi.org/10.1210/er.2015-1080

J Sex Med. Author manuscript; available in PMC 2009 Jun 30.Published in final edited form as: J Sex Med. 2008 Sep; 5(9): 2111–2118. Published online 2008 Jul 4. doi: 10.1111/j.1743-6109.2008.00922.x

Jung, C. and Inder, W. (2008). Management of adrenal insufficiency during the stress of medical illness and surgery. [online] Australasian Medical Publishing Company.www.mja.com.au/journal/2008/188/7/manageme

nt-adrenal-insufficiency-during-stress-medical-illness-and-surgery

Collard MD, C., Saatee, M.D, S., Reidy, M.D, A. and Liu, M.D, M. (2017). Perioperative Steroid Management: Approaches Based on Current Evidence. [online] Anesthesiology: Trusted Evidence Discovery in Practice. https://anesthesiology.pubs.asahq.org/article.aspx?articleid =2626031

Cortisol Pumping Survey
adrenalalternatives.com. (2020). Cortisol Pumping Survey. [online]https://docs.google.com/forms/d/1eWYZjIFP9HRJ DosvdimJnOr8p54Rmpx_2A4Xz40f77A/edit#responses

Notes: